Natural Product for Every Day:

Top 30 Effective Homemade Anti-Aging Remedies to Reverse the Aging Process

Table of content

Table of content 4

Introduction 6

Chapter 1 – 5 Homemade Natural Moisturizers 8

Deep Moisturizing Cream 8

All Natural Moisturizing Lotion 10

Homemade Facial Moisturizer...12

All Natural Vitamin E Skin Moisturizer...................................13

Homemade Anti-Aging Skin Cream 15

Chapter 2 – 5 DIY All-Natural Eye Cream/Lotions 17

Rosehip and Honey Eye Cream 17

DIY Homemade Eye Cream 18

Green Tea Anti-Aging Dark Circle Cream.................................20

Caffeine Eye Cream 21

Skin Firming Eye Serum 23

Chapter 3 – 5 DIY Wrinkle Creams 25

Frankincense Anti-Aging Wrinkle Cream 25

DIY Anti-Aging Wrinkle Cream 26

DIY Face Lift DMAE Wrinkle Cream..28

Anti-Aging Wrinkle Serum...29

Organic Honey Infused Wrinkle Fighter 31

Chapter 4 – 5 Natural Anti-Aging Facials and Masks................33

Homemade Anti-Aging Organic Facial....................................33

Skin Tightening and Pore Refining Facial 34

Carrot and Yogurt Anti-Aging Mask 36

Avocado Seed Anti-Aging Facial 37

Anti-Aging All Natural Clay Mask 38

Chapter 6 – 5 Smoothies to Reverse the Aging Process............40

Berry Blast Wrinkle Buster 41

The Lean Green Smoothie 42

Beautiful Youthful Skin Smoothie 44

Beauty and Vigor Smoothie 45

Turn Back Time Smoothie 46

Conclusion 48

FREE Bonus Reminder 49

Introduction

After trying just about every anti-aging product on the market, many people turn to all-natural, DIY anti-aging products. The high price of over the counter items is enough reason to give DIY a try. Most of the ingredients in these preparations and smoothies are all-natural and easy to find in the grocery store.

Many of these products contain essential oils. These oils can be found online for a modest price and a little goes a long way. Essential oils have enjoyed popularity in recent years as people discovered the awesome health and beauty properties of these oils. Today, essential oils are used in everything from homemade bath products to anti-aging hair and body preparations.

All the ingredients, including the essential oils, have been chosen for their particular expertise in anti-aging and health supporting benefits. Each recipe explains how to create the product, how it is used, and the benefits it provides. There are enough choices in this book to satisfy everyone who wants to give all-natural remedies a try.

This book delivers everything you need to get you on the road to health and beauty bliss. There is no need to acquire other books about all natural ingredients and their uses, it is all covered here. All of the products are among the best available for youthful beauty and health. Once you start creating your own beauty and health products you will end up spoiled by the low-cost choices that are now available to you.

If you find in the store, chances are, you can make it at home. Most over the counter products contain fillers, emulsifiers, and other additives to give the product a certain consistency and texture that can be achieved without the additives at home. In most cases, it is the additives that cause allergic reactions to the products; DIY products don't contain those additives so allergic reaction is not as prevalent.

With the recipes in this book you can create awesome eye creams that do eliminate circles, puffiness, and fine lines and wrinkles. The anti-aging facials and masks give your skin a healthy glow, deliver a powerhouse punch of skin and pore tightening while soothing and smoothing all skin types. Many of the ingredients in the products are edible, that's natural if you ask me.

You can even customize the scent and consistency of your creams, lotions, smoothies and masks by changing up the ingredients. You will begin to prefer certain ingredients. Once you understand their health and beauty properties you will be able to personalize the recipes to suit your taste.

Chapter 1 – 5 Homemade Natural Moisturizers

Deep Moisturizing Cream

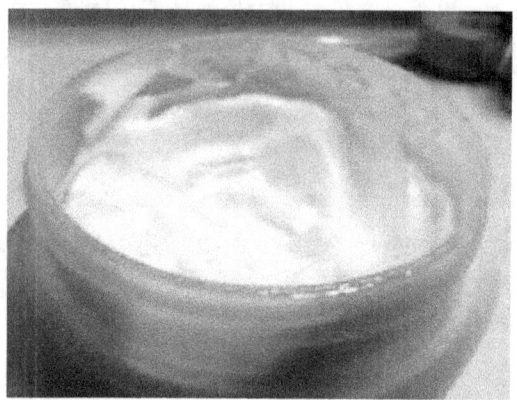

https://commons.wikimedia.org/wiki/File:Cold_Cream-2.jpg

Ingredients

½ cup of unrefined shea butter – Shea butter is a natural moisturizer with excellent nourishing properties. Using shea butter regularly has many benefits for aging skin; it is a natural anti-inflammatory thanks to cinnamic acids, and it contains organic compounds that repair damaged skin.

2 tbs of almond oil – Other oils can be used such as coconut oil, but almond oil is rich in vitamin E which supports healthy skin cell reproduction.

10 drops lavender essential oil – Lavender oil antiseptic and anti-inflammatory properties

5 drops rosemary essential oil – This essential oil provides antioxidants

3 drops carrot seed oil – Contains nutrients that rejuvenate and tighten the skin

Directions

Melt the shea butter in a pot over a low flame/heat once the shea is melted, add the almond oil and mix, then remove from the heat.

Pour the mix into a bowl and place it in the refrigerator for 15-20 minutes until it becomes solid. Once the mixture is solid it is time to add in the essential oils and the carrot seed oil. Use a mixer with a whisk and whip for about a minute or until the mix looks like whip cream. Put the cream in a jar and store it at room temperature.

Uses and Benefits

This deep moisturizer can be used all over including the face and hands. The natural shea butter and almond oil are humectants that moisturize and keep the skin hydrated. This cream relieves puffiness by reducing swelling, can be rubbed into joints to ease swelling, and it rejuvenates and tightens skin.

All Natural Moisturizing Lotion

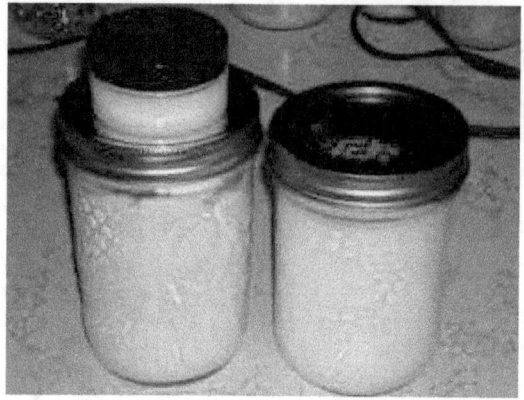

Ingredients

1 tbs of grated and packed beeswax – Softens and protects skin from environmental damage

1 tbs of unrefined shea butter

1/2 cup of avocado oil – This oil has a high concentration of vitamin E that can be absorbed through the skin

1 cup of water

Directions

Boil the water then put it aside

While the water is coming to a boil, melt the shea butter and beeswax in a double boiler (a stainless-steel bowl place into a pot of boiling water) when the shea butter and beeswax is melted it is time to add the avocado oil. Once all the ingredients are completely melted put the pot aside and once the water is hot but not scalding add the oil mix to the water and place it in a jar.

Using an immersion blender (a blender wand or blender stick) blend the mixture at the bottom for about 30 seconds then move the blender up and down until the entire mixture is emulsified (is not separating like oil and water). Repeat this process every 5 minutes until the mixture cools to room temperature.

Uses and Benefits

This all natural moisturizing lotion is superior to many over the counter lotions because it has natural concentrations of vitamin E and the smoothing and protection properties of beeswax helps to hold the moisture in place.

This natural moisturizer can be applied all over including the face. Apply after a bath or shower and before bed.

Homemade Facial Moisturizer

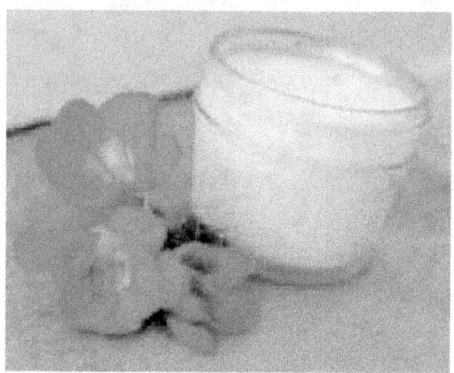

https://www.flickr.com/photos/64636759@N07/8690879244

Ingredients

1 tbs of Aloe Vera Gel – Aloe Vera calms and soothes damaged skin while providing healing properties

1 tsp of Vitamin E oil – Vitamin E fights free radicals with antioxidants

1 tsp of Jojoba oil – This oil contains antibacterial properties that supports skin cell production on damaged skin and it contains vitamins E and B which are essential to healthy skin

2 drops of Lavender Essential Oil

1 tbs of Coconut Oil – Coconut oil is a superior moisturizer for all skin types

Directions

Mix the Aloe Vera Gel, Jojoba Oil, and Coconut Oil together by hand, no blender/ mixer and add the lavender oil and mix until it is blended then store the cream in a small container and keep refrigerated. The cream will last up to six months in the refrigerator.

Uses and Benefits

This diy facial moisturizer provides antibacterial properties that make it a great choice for moisturizing skin that is prone to breakouts or eczema. The extra vitamin E and added vitamin B nourish the skin while moisturizing.

This facial moisturizer should be applied to the face in the morning and at night before bed.

All Natural Vitamin E Skin Moisturizer

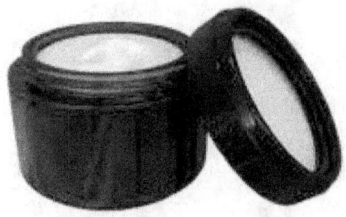

Ingredients

3 tbs cocoa butter – This butter is a superior moisturizer that penetrates the skin readily at room temperature and it provides deep moisturization to the skin

4 tbs coconut oil

1 tsp vitamin E oil

4 drops of lavender oil

Directions

In a double-boiler, or a heat-safe bowl over a pot of boiling water, melt the cocoa butter and coconut oil. Whisk together to combine.

Remove from heat and let cool slightly. Whisk in vitamin E oil and essential oil.

If you were using a pot, transfer your mixture to a medium-size bowl. Place the bowl, covered with plastic wrap, in the refrigerator for one hour.

Then, whisk vigorously until the cream is light and fluffy. This is easiest done with an electric mixer but I managed whisking by hand so you can do it that way too!

Cover bowl with plastic wrap again and refrigerate for half an hour.

Whisk vigorously again until light and fluffy. Scoop into a quarter-pint size mason jar and cover tightly.

Uses and Benefits

This awesome smelling vitamin E moisturizer provides nourishing vitamin E that protects and promotes healthy skin production. The anti-inflammatory properties of lavender add a skin soothing effect that make this moisturizer perfect for use in any skin care regimen.

Apply this moisturizer to clean skin before bed and in the morning as part of your skin care regimen.

Homemade Anti-Aging Skin Cream

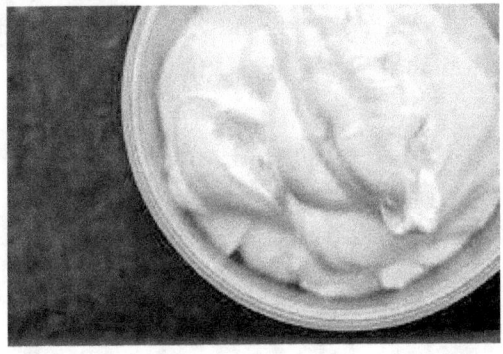

https://www.flickr.com/photos/46722918@N08/8498011657

Ingredients

1/3 cup of coconut oil

1 1/2 tbs of coconut butter grated

2 1/2 tsp of almond oil

10 drops of Tea Tree

7 drops of lavender essential oil

4 oz. canning jars

Directions

Place all ingredients in a bowl and mix with a whisk on high until the mixture is smooth and creamy then put it in a four-ounce canning jar.

Uses and Benefits

Use all over the body and face. The healing properties and superior moisturizing effects of the oils help the skin defy the signs of aging by softening the skin and repairing damage from daily life.

Chapter 2 – 5 DIY All-Natural Eye Cream/Lotions

Rosehip and Honey Eye Cream

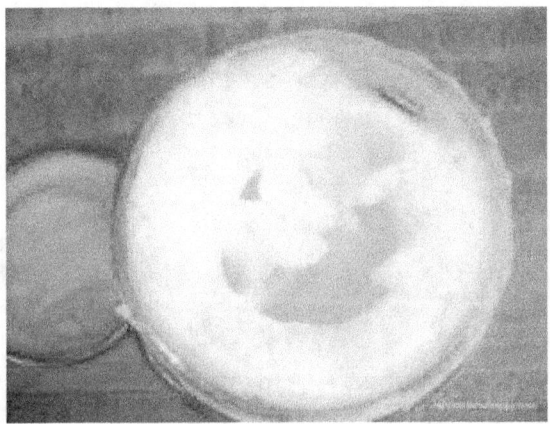

https://www.flickr.com/photos/39794839@N03/4819442821

Ingredients

6 tbs of avocado oil

2 tbs of beeswax

1/2 tbs of raw honey – Raw honey is full of antioxidants and it is widely known to slow down the effects of aging, it has proven antibacterial and healing properties.

2 tbs of rosehip seed oil – Provides vitamin c which has strong anti-aging properties and it is rich in omega 3, 6, and 9 fatty acids that heal and repair skin. It also provides sun protection.

3 drops of lavender essential oil

Directions

Using a double boiler, combine the beeswax and avocado oil and melt, then remove from the boiler and let it cool down a bit.

Add the raw honey and stir until completely blended then add the rosehip oil and the lavender oil and stir until the mixture is well blended and no longer separates then place the mixture into small jars or containers. Store the cream in a cool, dry place and it should last for at least 4 months

Uses and Benefits

Rosehip and honey eye cream is packed with anti-aging vitamins and nutrients, using it daily can reduce the signs of aging around the eyes as well as reduce redness, puffiness, while supporting the regeneration of healthy new skin cells.

Use it around the eyes daily, once in the morning under makeup and at night before bed.

DIY Homemade Eye Cream

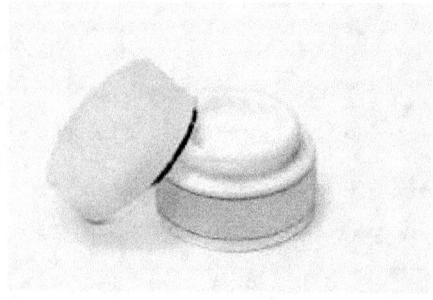

https://pixabay.com/en/photos/lid/

Ingredients

1/2 cup of coconut oil

6-8 Vitamin E capsules opened

10 drops Frankincense essential oil – This essential oil rejuvenates skin and gets rid of the fine lines and wrinkles.

Directions

Pour the coconut oil into a small container and microwave it for 15 seconds then pour the oil into a container you are going to use for storage. Open the vitamin E capsules and empty the liquid into the oil, then add the Frankincense oil and stir.

Put the container in the refrigerator until it solidifies, then you can keep it anywhere, this cream will not go bad.

Uses and Benefits

This cream is fabulous for removing makeup, it removes the makeup and leaves the skin around the eyes soft and beautiful. Use as an eye cream before bed and in the morning under makeup.

Green Tea Anti-Aging Dark Circle Cream

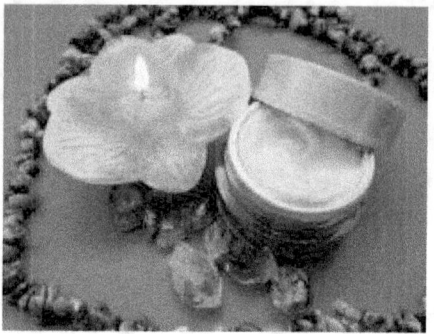

https://pixabay.com/en/skincare-cream-balm-candle-1122666/

Ingredients

2 tbs of almond oil

1 tbs of shea butter

3/4 tsp of beeswax

1 green tea bag -

2 drops of vitamin E oil

5 drops of peppermint essential oil – Peppermint has a cooling effect on skin that tightens the pores and the skin itself.

Directions

In a double boiler, melt the shea butter, vitamin E oil, shea butter, and beeswax. When the oils are melted pour the contents of the green tea bag into the oil and let the mixture sit over a low heat for 20 minutes in the double boiler, then pour the oil through a strainer and strain out the tea. Add the peppermint oil and mix until the entire mixture is well combined.

Pour the mix into a container with a lid then let it reach room temperature before using.

Uses and Benefits

Apply this cream using your ring finger so you are not pressing too hard on the delicate skin around the eyes. Using this cream under makeup and before bed will brighten the skin under the eyes and make dark circles a thing of the past... while moisturizing and tightening your skin.

Caffeine Eye Cream

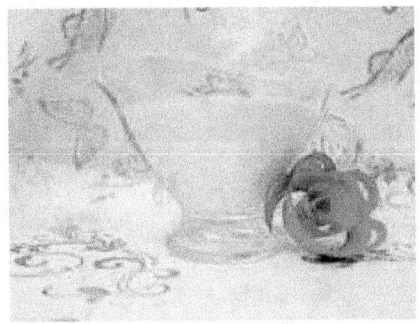

https://pixabay.com/en/lotion-skin-care-natural-spa-1244321/

Ingredients

1/4 cup of beeswax

1/4 cup coffee infused oil – Caffeine tightens skin and pores while invigorating by increasing circulation to the surface of the skin.

1/4 cup coconut oil

1 teaspoon jojoba oil

3 capsules vitamin E

5 drops chamomile essential oil – Chamomile oil calms and soothes while providing healing and antimicrobial properties.

Melt the beeswax in a double boiler over low heat and when it is melted add the coffee oil, jojoba, coconut, and vitamin e oils and stir. Remove from heat once the mixture is well combined and add the chamomile oil and mix.

Place the finished cream into a lidded container and keep it in the refrigerator.

Uses and Benefits

Caffeine eye cream delivers excellent skin tightening and refined pores while calming, soothing, moisturizing and repairing tired, aging, or damaged skin.

Apply under the eyes by dabbing, no rubbing, the skin around the eyes is delicate. Use this cream under makeup, before bed, or any other time your eyes look tired to brighten and tighten.

Skin Firming Eye Serum

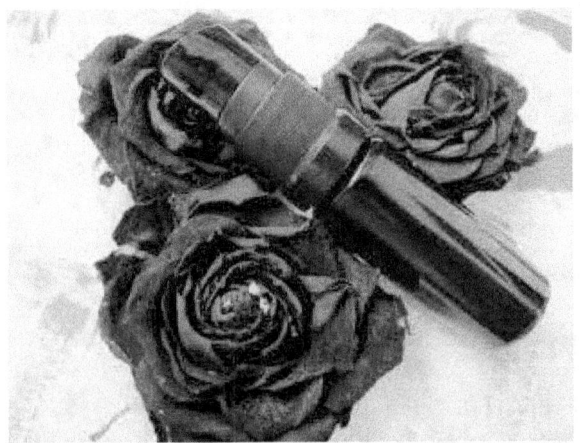

https://pixabay.com/en/serum-skin-care-luxury-cosmetic-1050959/

Ingredients

1 tbs of organic ground coffee

1 tbs of rosehip oil

1 tbs of argan oil -This wonder oil contains linoleic acid, omega 6, and antioxidants that fight fine lines. It is also a great moisturizer because it absorbs into the skin quickly and efficiently.

1/2 tbs of sea buckthorn oil – Sea buckthorn oil contains a huge number of antioxidants, it is one of the only plant sources of omega 3, 6, 9, and 7. It fights all the signs of aging and delivers protective moisture to the skin.

1/2 tbs jojoba oil

Directions

Put all the ingredients into a small glass jar and mix it well, make sure all the ingredients are well combined then place the jar in the sun, a windowsill is great for this, and leave it for 7 days.

After 7 days, use cheese cloth to strain out the grounds then pour the serum into a glass bottle with a lid.

Uses and Benefits

This eye serum has excellent anti-aging properties that fight fine lines and support healthy skin rejuvenation. The moisturizers and antioxidants in this serum will protect and moisturize the delicate area around the eyes.

Use this serum every morning after cleansing and before applying makeup.

Chapter 3 – 5 DIY Wrinkle Creams

Frankincense Anti-Aging Wrinkle Cream

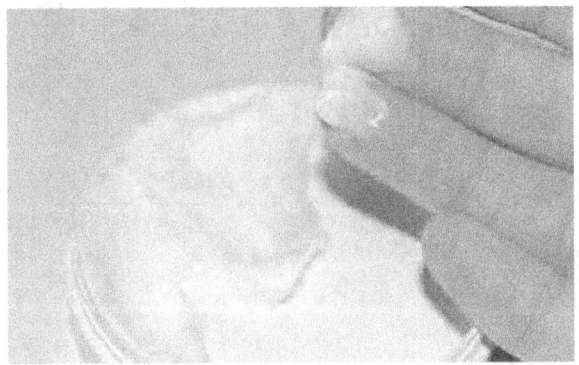

https://pixabay.com/en/cream-lubricate-the-cream-care-621340/

Ingredients

1/4 cup unrefined shea butter

1/4 cup coconut oil

10 drops of frankincense essential oil

7 drops of lavender essential oil

Directions

Melt the shea butter and coconut oil in a double boiler and stir until well blended then remove from the heat and let it cool down for 30 minutes.

Add frankincense and lavender oils and stir until the mixture is well blended. Set the mix aside or place in the refrigerator until it is solidified then using a mixer, whip the mix until it has the consistency of butter.

Put into a four-ounce mason jar. This cream will last for about 6 months, there is no need to refrigerate.

Uses and Benefits

This wrinkle cream delivers fantastic reduction in the everyday signs of aging. It reduces fine lines and moisturizes while tightening the skin. Use this cream all over including the face at least once a day.

DIY Anti-Aging Wrinkle Cream

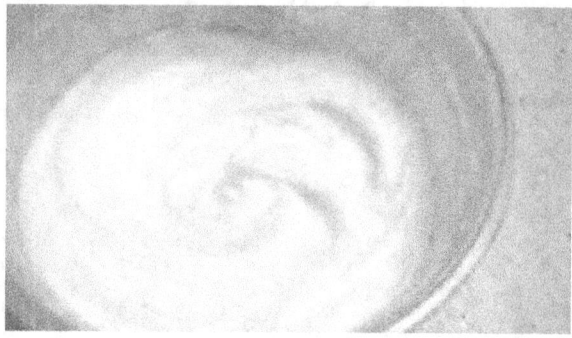

https://www.flickr.com/photos/ecokaren/6554283227

Ingredients

¼ cup almond oil

2 tablespoons coconut oil

2 tablespoons beeswax

½ teaspoon vitamin E oil

1 tablespoon shea butter

A few drops of your favorite essential oil to customize

Directions

Put the ingredients in a glass jar, do not put a lid on it and place it in a pot of water and bring the water to a simmer and when the ingredients begin to melt, stir.

When the mix is well blended pour it into a glass jar and let it sit until it solidifies then put the lid on and store in a cool, dry place.

Uses and Benefits

This anti-aging wrinkle cream fights lines and wrinkles, protects skin from environmental contaminants, smooths and moisturizes while delivering support for healthy skin cell rejuvenation.

Use this cream every time you wash. It can be used on all parts of the body but the main use is to reduce lines and wrinkles on the face.

DIY Face Lift DMAE Wrinkle Cream

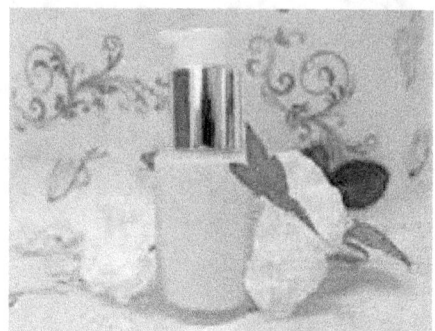

https://pixabay.com/en/skin-care-cosmetics-natural-1309504/

Ingredients

1/4 cup of shea butter

1 tbs of coconut oil

1 tsp of almond oil

8 drops of frankincense

8 drops of lemon oil – Lemon oil tightens and rejuvenates tired saggy skin. It also delivers a brightening effect to dull skin or dark circles.

8 drops of lavender

1 Capsule DMAE – DMAE is a supplement that can be purchased in health stores. DMAE is used in many expensive and potent over the counter wrinkle creams.

Few drops of distilled water – open the DMAE capsule and combine the water and the powder, mix until the DMAE and water are completely blended.

Directions

Melt the shea butter and coconut oil in a double boiler. Once the mixture is liquid remove it from the heat.

Add the almond oil and the essential oils into the mix and stir until well blended then allow the mixture to solidify in the refrigerator for 20 minutes.

Once the mixture solidifies, use a mixer and whip the mix until it is the consistency of frosting.

Put the mixture to a four-ounce. glass jar.

Uses and Benefits

Use this cream every time you wash, apply to all areas where you want to fight the fine lines and wrinkles of aging. The DMAE in this diy cream will deliver results you can see after using it for at least a week.

Anti-Aging Wrinkle Serum

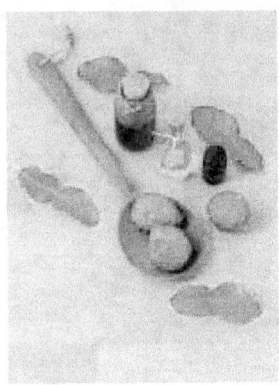

Ingredients

2 tbs of rosehip oil

2 tbs of almond Oil

10 drops of cypress essential oil -

10 drops of geranium essential oil -

7 drops of frankincense essential oil

Directions

Mix and blend all ingredients until completely combined and place the serum in a bottle with a lid.

Uses and Benefits

Use this serum at night to wake with visible bright and soft skin. A small amount will go a long way, too much will create a greasy film. This is an easy product to make and it the benefits of skin tightening, brightening, and the reduction in fine lines and wrinkles is truly amazing.

Organic Honey Infused Wrinkle Fighter

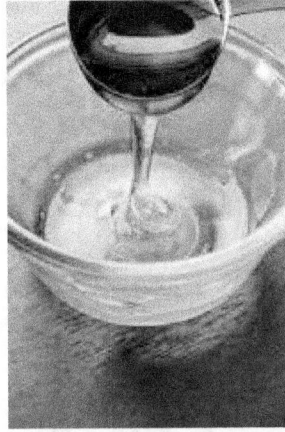

https://pixabay.com/en/honey-ingredient-healthy-food-1460406/

Ingredients

1 egg yolk

2 table spoons of almond oil

1/2 teaspoon of raw organic honey

3 teaspoons of coconut oil

Directions

Mix all ingredients together and continue mixing until the mixture is well blended and has a smooth consistency.

Pour the mixture into a glass container and keep it in the refrigerator so it will remain fresh.

Uses and Benefits

Apply a small amount of this serum to the face after washing and a least two hours before going to bed. The serum is thick and rich, too much will create a thick layer on the skin that will take a long time to absorb so remove any excess with a soft cotton pad. This serum will give you a beautiful complexion while reducing fine lines and wrinkles and moisturizing skin all day.

Chapter 4 – 5 Natural Anti-Aging Facials and Masks

Homemade Anti-Aging Organic Facial

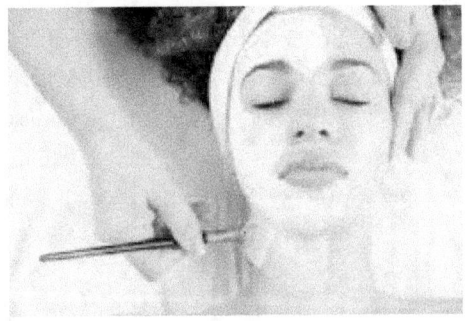

https://www.flickr.com/photos/93609956@N05/9509632741

Ingredients

1 egg yolk

2 teaspoons of raw honey

½ teaspoon of unflavored gelatin

1 teaspoon of lemon juice

2 drops frankincense essential oil

2 drops lavender essential oil

Directions

Use a whisk and whip all the ingredients until the mixture is well blended then put the mix into a container

Uses and Benefits

Wash your face and leave it wet, then apply the mask to your damp/wet face. Cover all areas of the face and allow it to sit until it is tight and dry on your face then wash it off and pat dry. Repeat the application of this mask 2 times a week to benefit from all the anti-aging properties this mask has. Keep the unused portion in the refrigerator and take it out and let it reach room temperature before using.

Skin Tightening and Pore Refining Facial

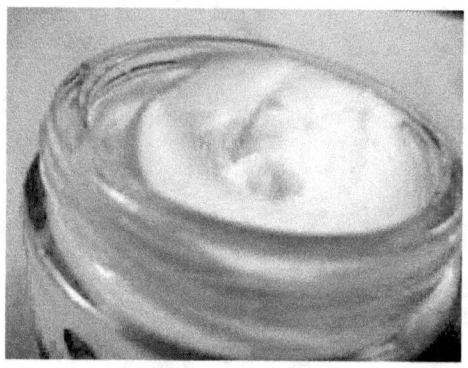

https://www.flickr.com/photos/sunshinecity/786584004

Ingredients

Half a cucumber with the skin on

1 egg white

Some cornstarch

2 drops of frankincense oil

Directions

Using a blender, whip the cucumber and egg whites until there is a froth, then pour it into a glass jar and add the frankincense. Add cornstarch slowly while mixing, use enough cornstarch in the mix to create a paste consistency.

Uses and Benefits

Before applying the mask, massage the face to increase blood flow to the surface of the skin.

Wet your face with warm water and apply the mask to all areas and leave the mask in place for 15 minutes then rinse and dry.

It is a good idea to use some witch hazel as an astringent, witch hazel is gentle to the skin and it will tighten the skin and pores even more.

This mask reduces the appearance of large pores or sagging skin by tightening both and providing essential vitamins to the skin for healthy skin cell production. It also removes impurities from the skin and reduces lines and wrinkles.

Carrot and Yogurt Anti-Aging Mask

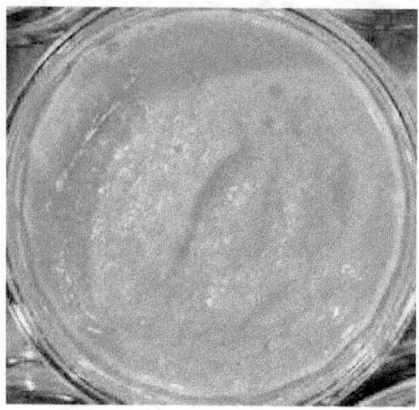

https://pixabay.com/en/photos/an%20avocado/

Ingredients

1 tbs of cornstarch

5 tbs of pureed carrot

1 tbs of yogurt

water

Directions

Combine the carrot and yogurt in a glass jar and mix until the mixture is completely blended, add the cornstarch and enough water to create a creamy consistency.

Uses and Benefits

This mask delivers antioxidants, vitamins, and moisture to tired, overworked skin. Yogurt tightens and softens the skin and the carrot delivers the antioxidant boost that fights the lines and wrinkles.

Cover your entire face with this mask and leave it on for at least 15 minutes then use warm water to wash it off. When you remove the mask your skin will have a youthful, healthy glow, and sagging skin will be firmer and suppler.

Avocado Seed Anti-Aging Facial

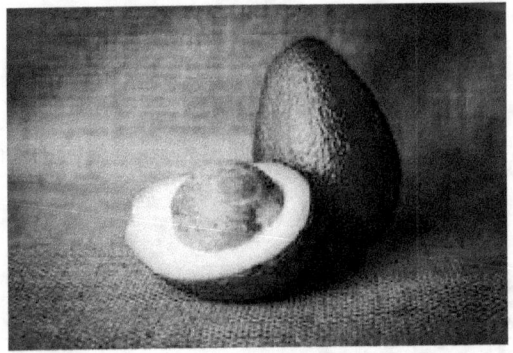

https://pixabay.com/en/avocado-vegetable-cut-half-pit-933060/

Ingredients

1 egg white – Tightens skin and pores while making skin smooth and soft

2 tsp Avocado seed powder – This powder contains antioxidants that repair cell damage and help skin replace old cells with new.

Directions

Beat the egg white until it forms peaks, just like whipped cream then add 2 teaspoons of avocado seed powder, mix together until blended.

Uses and Benefits

As soon as you complete the facial mix, apply it to your face and neck. Cover all areas of the face and neck including under and around the eyes. Leave the mix to harden on your face for 20 minutes, then using warm water, wash it off and pat your skin dry.

The awesome antioxidants in the facial not only tighten and firm, they nourish, smooth, and repair the skin. Repeat this facial at least once a week for continued results.

Anti-Aging All Natural Clay Mask

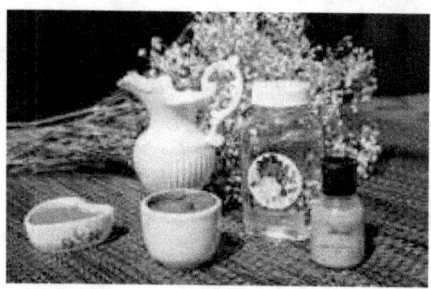

https://pixabay.com/en/mask-facial-mud-water-of-roses-spa-1231843/

Ingredients

4 teaspoons of filtered water

1 teaspoon of raw honey

1 drop of frankincense oil

1 drop of lemon essential oil

2 drops of rosehip essential oil

2 teaspoons of bentonite clay

2 teaspoons of kelp powder

Directions

Mix together the water, raw honey, and essential oils in a plastic bowl or container, the container must be plastic because the clay will react to metal. Mix until completely blended.

Add the bentonite clay and kelp powder and continue mixing with a wooden or plastic utensil, add more water to create a consistency that will go on smoothly.

Uses and Benefits

Apply the mask to your face and neck avoiding the eye area. Let the mask dry and after 10 minutes rinse it off with warm water and pat dry.

Your skin will look soft and smooth, fine lines and wrinkles will be less obvious because this mask tightens and nourishes the skin. Use this mask weekly to see consistent results. The more you stick to a routine with this mask, the better your skin will become.

Chapter 6 – 5 Smoothies to Reverse the Aging Process

Everyone knows the benefits of juicing; you get all the benefits of the veggies and fruits, concentrated into a single glass of juice. Well there is another way to get some awesome age reversing results without a juicer; you can just use your blender! These smoothies are packed with everything you need to fight the aging process and win. Best of all, smoothies are awesome tasting and easy to make.

It doesn't matter which smoothie you choose, these smoothies provide concentrated antioxidants, vitamins, and nutrients, that provide your body with what it needs to feel younger and stay active. Each smoothie delivers potent and proven age fighting nutrients your body will love. These delicious drinks will do more than support beautiful skin; they fight inflammation and boost the immune system.

Berry Blast Wrinkle Buster

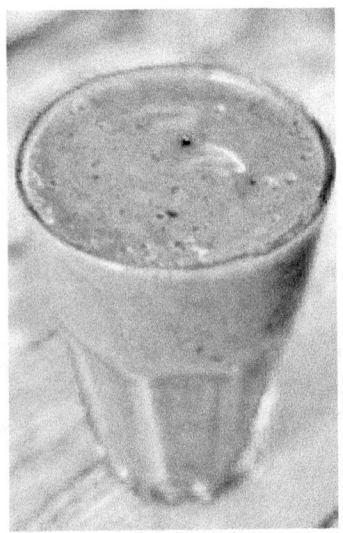

https://www.flickr.com/photos/anne-cathrine_nyberg/7189773492

Ingredients

1½ cups of cold coconut water

2 cups of chopped up kale

2 cups of blueberries frozen

½ an orange peeled

1 tbs of flax seeds

2 chopped brazil nuts

Directions

Put all the ingredients into a blender and blend until the smoothie is well blended.

Benefits

The coconut water delivers antioxidants, vitamins, minerals, and it is low in calories. Kale provides fiber and to aid in digestion and it is packed with vitamins and minerals. The blueberries are a super food, full of antioxidants and vitamins and the orange adds vitamin c for a strong immune system. Brazil nuts have protein, and potassium among other super minerals while flax seeds deliver omega 3's and antioxidants.

The Lean Green Smoothie

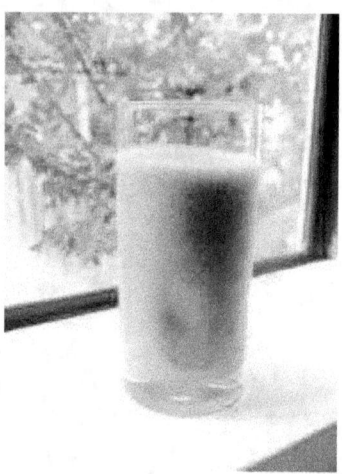

https://commons.wikimedia.org/wiki/File:Green_Smoothie_(3652108873).jpg

Ingredients

1 cup of spinach

1/2 of a medium banana

2 tbs of avocado

1 tbs of sunflower seeds

2 tbs of lemon juice

1 cup of almond milk unsweetened

Directions

Put all the ingredients into a blender and blend until the mixture is smooth.

Benefits

Avocados can lower triglycerides and they pack more potassium than a banana all while delivering some omega fatty acids. Spinach provides much needed protein, vitamin B6 and a host of other vitamins that support healthy muscles including the heart. Bananas are a good source of potassium which is essential to heart health. Sunflower seeds are an awesome source of vitamin e and healthy fats, lemon juice boosts the immune system with some extra vitamin c and unsweetened almond milk adds more potassium, calcium, and vitamin E.

Beautiful Youthful Skin Smoothie

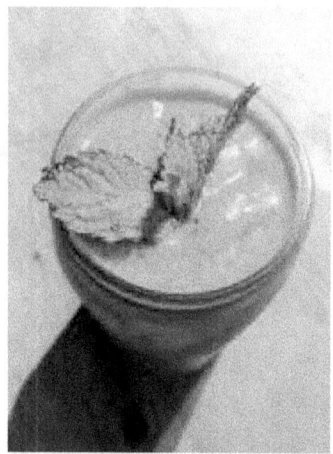

https://en.wikipedia.org/wiki/Smoothie

Ingredients

One orange peeled

1 medium banana peeled

½ cup of frozen blueberries

½ cup of fat-free yogurt, plain

2 tablespoons of chia seeds

1 tablespoon of agave nectar

¼ cup of frozen strawberries

Directions

Put the ingredients into your blender and blend until it is smooth and well mixed

Benefits

Antioxidants are some of the best wrinkle fighters around and this smoothie is packed to the brim with them. Fiber, protein, and omega fatty acids are found in chia seeds, these essential nutrients are heart healthy, muscle healthy, brain healthy, and they are just great for skin. Agave nectar is a great alternative for sugar to sweeten things up and the yogurt provides good bacteria for the gut. The high vitamin c content of oranges provides immune boosting properties to this already super healthy, rejuvenating smoothie.

Beauty and Vigor Smoothie

Ingredients

1/2 cup of strawberries frozen

1/2 cup of mixed berries frozen

¼ cup of sesame seeds

1 tbs of honey

1/2 cup of orange juice

Some ice cubes

Directions

Blend all the ingredients together in a blender until it reaches the consistency you are after. Too much blending will oxidize some of the ingredients and it will lose nutrients, so don't blend too long.

Benefits

The berries provide the antioxidant properties for younger looking skin, the sesame seeds deliver calcium, vitamin b6, and protein which all contribute to a healthy immune system as well as energy. The orange juice provides vitamin c for energy and a healthy immune system and the honey has flavonoids that have properties that protect against cancer, along with more antioxidants to make this drink a power house of energy, health, and beauty.

Turn Back Time Smoothie

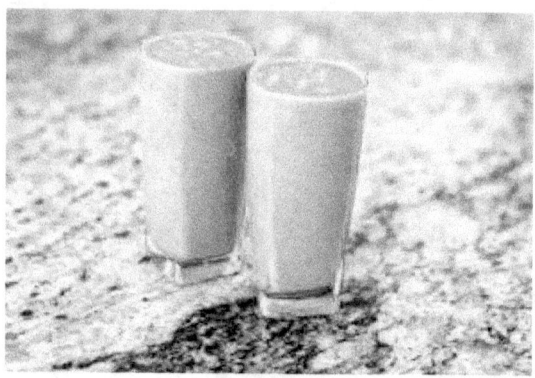

https://pixabay.com/en/photos/nutrients/

Ingredients

1 1/2 cups of frozen pineapples

1 cup of frozen mangoes

1 cup of frozen chopped kale

1 cup of coconut water

2 tablespoons of hemp seed powder

Directions

Blend all the ingredients together in a blender and blend until it reaches your desired consistency.

Benefits

Pineapples are an awesome healthy addition to any smoothie, they provide soluble and insoluble fiber, and among a slew of excellent vitamins and minerals they deliver beta-carotene for healthy skin and eyes. Mangoes have a bunch of vitamins and minerals and these too deliver beta-carotene for skin and eyes. Omega 3 and 6 for heart and circulatory health are found in hemp seed powder and chopped kale and coconut water provide antioxidants, vitamins, and minerals for immune support and youthful skin.

Conclusion

The all natural and homemade anti-aging products you have learned to create and use are also a great gift idea. With all the great creams, serums, and smoothies you know how to make, you can put together an awesome basket of beauty for friends and family. It will make them happy and save you a ton of cash!

Looking and feeling your best is worth the small amount of effort used to create these wonderful all natural products. No more burning skin because something in the anti-wrinkle cream is irritating, and there is less chance of an allergic reaction when you know every ingredient used.

Get out and enjoy your new-found energy and show off your beautiful skin. when someone asks you how you stay looking and feeling so young; tell them the answer is in the refrigerator not the beauty supply store!

FREE Bonus Reminder

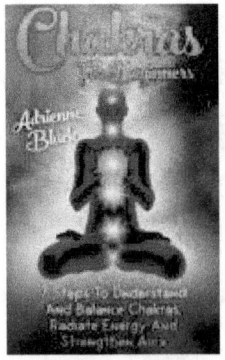

If you have not grabbed it yet, please go ahead and download your special bonus E book *"Chakras for Beginners. 7 Steps To Understand And Balance Chakras, Radiate Energy, And Strengthen Aura"*.

Simply Click the Button Below

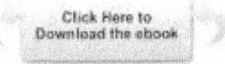

OR Go to This Page

http://lifehacksworld.com/free

BONUS #2: More Free & Discounted Books & Products

Do you want to receive more Free/Discounted Books or Products?

We have a mailing list where we send out our new Books or Products when they go free or with a discount on Amazon. Click on the link below to sign up for Free & Discount Book & Product Promotions.

=> Sign Up for Free & Discount Book & Product Promotions <=

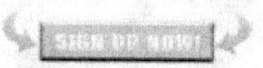

OR Go to this URL

http://zbit.ly/1WBb1Ek

www.ingramcontent.com/pod-product-compliance
Lightning Source LLC
Chambersburg PA
CBHW071136280526
45787CB00003B/1301